This

Daily Nutrition

Logbook

belongs to:

_____

_____

_____

from _____ to _____

Date:

Breakfast

Time	Item	Servings	Calories	Sugar	Protein	Fat	Carbs

Lunch

Time	Item	Servings	Calories	Sugar	Protein	Fat	Carbs

Dinner

Time	Item	Servings	Calories	Sugar	Protein	Fat	Carbs

Snacks

Time	Item	Servings	Calories	Sugar	Protein	Fat	Carbs

Total:

Servings	Calories	Sugar	Protein	Fat	Carbs

Date:

Breakfast

Time	Item	Servings	Calories	Sugar	Protein	Fat	Carbs

Lunch

Time	Item	Servings	Calories	Sugar	Protein	Fat	Carbs

Dinner

Time	Item	Servings	Calories	Sugar	Protein	Fat	Carbs

Snacks

Time	Item	Servings	Calories	Sugar	Protein	Fat	Carbs

Total:

Servings	Calories	Sugar	Protein	Fat	Carbs

Date:

Breakfast

Time	Item	Servings	Calories	Sugar	Protein	Fat	Carbs

Lunch

Time	Item	Servings	Calories	Sugar	Protein	Fat	Carbs

Dinner

Time	Item	Servings	Calories	Sugar	Protein	Fat	Carbs

Snacks

Time	Item	Servings	Calories	Sugar	Protein	Fat	Carbs

Total:

Servings	Calories	Sugar	Protein	Fat	Carbs

Date:

Breakfast

Time	Item	Servings	Calories	Sugar	Protein	Fat	Carbs

Lunch

Time	Item	Servings	Calories	Sugar	Protein	Fat	Carbs

Dinner

Time	Item	Servings	Calories	Sugar	Protein	Fat	Carbs

Snacks

Time	Item	Servings	Calories	Sugar	Protein	Fat	Carbs

Total:

Servings	Calories	Sugar	Protein	Fat	Carbs

Date:

Breakfast

Time	Item	Servings	Calories	Sugar	Protein	Fat	Carbs

Lunch

Time	Item	Servings	Calories	Sugar	Protein	Fat	Carbs

Dinner

Time	Item	Servings	Calories	Sugar	Protein	Fat	Carbs

Snacks

Time	Item	Servings	Calories	Sugar	Protein	Fat	Carbs

Total:

Servings	Calories	Sugar	Protein	Fat	Carbs

Date:

Breakfast

Time	Item	Servings	Calories	Sugar	Protein	Fat	Carbs

Lunch

Time	Item	Servings	Calories	Sugar	Protein	Fat	Carbs

Dinner

Time	Item	Servings	Calories	Sugar	Protein	Fat	Carbs

Snacks

Time	Item	Servings	Calories	Sugar	Protein	Fat	Carbs

Total:

Servings	Calories	Sugar	Protein	Fat	Carbs

Date:

Breakfast

Time	Item	Servings	Calories	Sugar	Protein	Fat	Carbs

Lunch

Time	Item	Servings	Calories	Sugar	Protein	Fat	Carbs

Dinner

Time	Item	Servings	Calories	Sugar	Protein	Fat	Carbs

Snacks

Time	Item	Servings	Calories	Sugar	Protein	Fat	Carbs

Total:

Servings	Calories	Sugar	Protein	Fat	Carbs

Date:

Breakfast

Time	Item	Servings	Calories	Sugar	Protein	Fat	Carbs

Lunch

Time	Item	Servings	Calories	Sugar	Protein	Fat	Carbs

Dinner

Time	Item	Servings	Calories	Sugar	Protein	Fat	Carbs

Snacks

Time	Item	Servings	Calories	Sugar	Protein	Fat	Carbs

Total:

Servings	Calories	Sugar	Protein	Fat	Carbs

Date:

Breakfast

Time	Item	Servings	Calories	Sugar	Protein	Fat	Carbs

Lunch

Time	Item	Servings	Calories	Sugar	Protein	Fat	Carbs

Dinner

Time	Item	Servings	Calories	Sugar	Protein	Fat	Carbs

Snacks

Time	Item	Servings	Calories	Sugar	Protein	Fat	Carbs

Total:

Servings	Calories	Sugar	Protein	Fat	Carbs

Date:

Breakfast

Time	Item	Servings	Calories	Sugar	Protein	Fat	Carbs

Lunch

Time	Item	Servings	Calories	Sugar	Protein	Fat	Carbs

Dinner

Time	Item	Servings	Calories	Sugar	Protein	Fat	Carbs

Snacks

Time	Item	Servings	Calories	Sugar	Protein	Fat	Carbs

Total:

Servings	Calories	Sugar	Protein	Fat	Carbs

Date:

Breakfast

Time	Item	Servings	Calories	Sugar	Protein	Fat	Carbs

Lunch

Time	Item	Servings	Calories	Sugar	Protein	Fat	Carbs

Dinner

Time	Item	Servings	Calories	Sugar	Protein	Fat	Carbs

Snacks

Time	Item	Servings	Calories	Sugar	Protein	Fat	Carbs

Total:

Servings	Calories	Sugar	Protein	Fat	Carbs

Date:

Breakfast

Time	Item	Servings	Calories	Sugar	Protein	Fat	Carbs

Lunch

Time	Item	Servings	Calories	Sugar	Protein	Fat	Carbs

Dinner

Time	Item	Servings	Calories	Sugar	Protein	Fat	Carbs

Snacks

Time	Item	Servings	Calories	Sugar	Protein	Fat	Carbs

Total:

Servings	Calories	Sugar	Protein	Fat	Carbs

Date:

Breakfast

Time	Item	Servings	Calories	Sugar	Protein	Fat	Carbs

Lunch

Time	Item	Servings	Calories	Sugar	Protein	Fat	Carbs

Dinner

Time	Item	Servings	Calories	Sugar	Protein	Fat	Carbs

Snacks

Time	Item	Servings	Calories	Sugar	Protein	Fat	Carbs

Total:

Servings	Calories	Sugar	Protein	Fat	Carbs

Date:

Breakfast

Time	Item	Servings	Calories	Sugar	Protein	Fat	Carbs

Lunch

Time	Item	Servings	Calories	Sugar	Protein	Fat	Carbs

Dinner

Time	Item	Servings	Calories	Sugar	Protein	Fat	Carbs

Snacks

Time	Item	Servings	Calories	Sugar	Protein	Fat	Carbs

Total:

Servings	Calories	Sugar	Protein	Fat	Carbs

Date:

Breakfast

Time	Item	Servings	Calories	Sugar	Protein	Fat	Carbs

Lunch

Time	Item	Servings	Calories	Sugar	Protein	Fat	Carbs

Dinner

Time	Item	Servings	Calories	Sugar	Protein	Fat	Carbs

Snacks

Time	Item	Servings	Calories	Sugar	Protein	Fat	Carbs

Total:

Servings	Calories	Sugar	Protein	Fat	Carbs

Date:

Breakfast

Time	Item	Servings	Calories	Sugar	Protein	Fat	Carbs

Lunch

Time	Item	Servings	Calories	Sugar	Protein	Fat	Carbs

Dinner

Time	Item	Servings	Calories	Sugar	Protein	Fat	Carbs

Snacks

Time	Item	Servings	Calories	Sugar	Protein	Fat	Carbs

Total:

Servings	Calories	Sugar	Protein	Fat	Carbs

Date:

Breakfast

Time	Item	Servings	Calories	Sugar	Protein	Fat	Carbs

Lunch

Time	Item	Servings	Calories	Sugar	Protein	Fat	Carbs

Dinner

Time	Item	Servings	Calories	Sugar	Protein	Fat	Carbs

Snacks

Time	Item	Servings	Calories	Sugar	Protein	Fat	Carbs

Total:

Servings	Calories	Sugar	Protein	Fat	Carbs

Date:

Breakfast

Time	Item	Servings	Calories	Sugar	Protein	Fat	Carbs

Lunch

Time	Item	Servings	Calories	Sugar	Protein	Fat	Carbs

Dinner

Time	Item	Servings	Calories	Sugar	Protein	Fat	Carbs

Snacks

Time	Item	Servings	Calories	Sugar	Protein	Fat	Carbs

Total:

Servings	Calories	Sugar	Protein	Fat	Carbs

Date:

Breakfast

Time	Item	Servings	Calories	Sugar	Protein	Fat	Carbs

Lunch

Time	Item	Servings	Calories	Sugar	Protein	Fat	Carbs

Dinner

Time	Item	Servings	Calories	Sugar	Protein	Fat	Carbs

Snacks

Time	Item	Servings	Calories	Sugar	Protein	Fat	Carbs

Total:

Servings	Calories	Sugar	Protein	Fat	Carbs

Date:

Breakfast

Time	Item	Servings	Calories	Sugar	Protein	Fat	Carbs

Lunch

Time	Item	Servings	Calories	Sugar	Protein	Fat	Carbs

Dinner

Time	Item	Servings	Calories	Sugar	Protein	Fat	Carbs

Snacks

Time	Item	Servings	Calories	Sugar	Protein	Fat	Carbs

Total:

Servings	Calories	Sugar	Protein	Fat	Carbs

Date:

Breakfast

Time	Item	Servings	Calories	Sugar	Protein	Fat	Carbs

Lunch

Time	Item	Servings	Calories	Sugar	Protein	Fat	Carbs

Dinner

Time	Item	Servings	Calories	Sugar	Protein	Fat	Carbs

Snacks

Time	Item	Servings	Calories	Sugar	Protein	Fat	Carbs

Total:

Servings	Calories	Sugar	Protein	Fat	Carbs

Date:

Breakfast

Time	Item	Servings	Calories	Sugar	Protein	Fat	Carbs

Lunch

Time	Item	Servings	Calories	Sugar	Protein	Fat	Carbs

Dinner

Time	Item	Servings	Calories	Sugar	Protein	Fat	Carbs

Snacks

Time	Item	Servings	Calories	Sugar	Protein	Fat	Carbs

Total:

Servings	Calories	Sugar	Protein	Fat	Carbs

Date:

Breakfast

Time	Item	Servings	Calories	Sugar	Protein	Fat	Carbs

Lunch

Time	Item	Servings	Calories	Sugar	Protein	Fat	Carbs

Dinner

Time	Item	Servings	Calories	Sugar	Protein	Fat	Carbs

Snacks

Time	Item	Servings	Calories	Sugar	Protein	Fat	Carbs

Total:

Servings	Calories	Sugar	Protein	Fat	Carbs

Date:

Breakfast

Time	Item	Servings	Calories	Sugar	Protein	Fat	Carbs

Lunch

Time	Item	Servings	Calories	Sugar	Protein	Fat	Carbs

Dinner

Time	Item	Servings	Calories	Sugar	Protein	Fat	Carbs

Snacks

Time	Item	Servings	Calories	Sugar	Protein	Fat	Carbs

Total:

Servings	Calories	Sugar	Protein	Fat	Carbs

Date:

Breakfast

Time	Item	Servings	Calories	Sugar	Protein	Fat	Carbs

Lunch

Time	Item	Servings	Calories	Sugar	Protein	Fat	Carbs

Dinner

Time	Item	Servings	Calories	Sugar	Protein	Fat	Carbs

Snacks

Time	Item	Servings	Calories	Sugar	Protein	Fat	Carbs

Total:

Servings	Calories	Sugar	Protein	Fat	Carbs

Date:

Breakfast

Time	Item	Servings	Calories	Sugar	Protein	Fat	Carbs

Lunch

Time	Item	Servings	Calories	Sugar	Protein	Fat	Carbs

Dinner

Time	Item	Servings	Calories	Sugar	Protein	Fat	Carbs

Snacks

Time	Item	Servings	Calories	Sugar	Protein	Fat	Carbs

Total:

Servings	Calories	Sugar	Protein	Fat	Carbs

Date:

Breakfast

Time	Item	Servings	Calories	Sugar	Protein	Fat	Carbs

Lunch

Time	Item	Servings	Calories	Sugar	Protein	Fat	Carbs

Dinner

Time	Item	Servings	Calories	Sugar	Protein	Fat	Carbs

Snacks

Time	Item	Servings	Calories	Sugar	Protein	Fat	Carbs

Total:

Servings	Calories	Sugar	Protein	Fat	Carbs

Date:

Breakfast

Time	Item	Servings	Calories	Sugar	Protein	Fat	Carbs

Lunch

Time	Item	Servings	Calories	Sugar	Protein	Fat	Carbs

Dinner

Time	Item	Servings	Calories	Sugar	Protein	Fat	Carbs

Snacks

Time	Item	Servings	Calories	Sugar	Protein	Fat	Carbs

Total:

Servings	Calories	Sugar	Protein	Fat	Carbs

Date:

Breakfast

Time	Item	Servings	Calories	Sugar	Protein	Fat	Carbs

Lunch

Time	Item	Servings	Calories	Sugar	Protein	Fat	Carbs

Dinner

Time	Item	Servings	Calories	Sugar	Protein	Fat	Carbs

Snacks

Time	Item	Servings	Calories	Sugar	Protein	Fat	Carbs

Total:

Servings	Calories	Sugar	Protein	Fat	Carbs

Date:

Breakfast

Time	Item	Servings	Calories	Sugar	Protein	Fat	Carbs

Lunch

Time	Item	Servings	Calories	Sugar	Protein	Fat	Carbs

Dinner

Time	Item	Servings	Calories	Sugar	Protein	Fat	Carbs

Snacks

Time	Item	Servings	Calories	Sugar	Protein	Fat	Carbs

Total:

Servings	Calories	Sugar	Protein	Fat	Carbs

Date:

Breakfast

Time	Item	Servings	Calories	Sugar	Protein	Fat	Carbs

Lunch

Time	Item	Servings	Calories	Sugar	Protein	Fat	Carbs

Dinner

Time	Item	Servings	Calories	Sugar	Protein	Fat	Carbs

Snacks

Time	Item	Servings	Calories	Sugar	Protein	Fat	Carbs

Total:

Servings	Calories	Sugar	Protein	Fat	Carbs

Date:

Breakfast

Time	Item	Servings	Calories	Sugar	Protein	Fat	Carbs

Lunch

Time	Item	Servings	Calories	Sugar	Protein	Fat	Carbs

Dinner

Time	Item	Servings	Calories	Sugar	Protein	Fat	Carbs

Snacks

Time	Item	Servings	Calories	Sugar	Protein	Fat	Carbs

Total:

Servings	Calories	Sugar	Protein	Fat	Carbs

Date:

Breakfast

Time	Item	Servings	Calories	Sugar	Protein	Fat	Carbs

Lunch

Time	Item	Servings	Calories	Sugar	Protein	Fat	Carbs

Dinner

Time	Item	Servings	Calories	Sugar	Protein	Fat	Carbs

Snacks

Time	Item	Servings	Calories	Sugar	Protein	Fat	Carbs

Total:

Servings	Calories	Sugar	Protein	Fat	Carbs

Date:

Breakfast

Time	Item	Servings	Calories	Sugar	Protein	Fat	Carbs

Lunch

Time	Item	Servings	Calories	Sugar	Protein	Fat	Carbs

Dinner

Time	Item	Servings	Calories	Sugar	Protein	Fat	Carbs

Snacks

Time	Item	Servings	Calories	Sugar	Protein	Fat	Carbs

Total:

Servings	Calories	Sugar	Protein	Fat	Carbs

Date:

Breakfast

Time	Item	Servings	Calories	Sugar	Protein	Fat	Carbs

Lunch

Time	Item	Servings	Calories	Sugar	Protein	Fat	Carbs

Dinner

Time	Item	Servings	Calories	Sugar	Protein	Fat	Carbs

Snacks

Time	Item	Servings	Calories	Sugar	Protein	Fat	Carbs

Total:

Servings	Calories	Sugar	Protein	Fat	Carbs

Date:

Breakfast

Time	Item	Servings	Calories	Sugar	Protein	Fat	Carbs

Lunch

Time	Item	Servings	Calories	Sugar	Protein	Fat	Carbs

Dinner

Time	Item	Servings	Calories	Sugar	Protein	Fat	Carbs

Snacks

Time	Item	Servings	Calories	Sugar	Protein	Fat	Carbs

Total:

Servings	Calories	Sugar	Protein	Fat	Carbs

Date:

Breakfast

Time	Item	Servings	Calories	Sugar	Protein	Fat	Carbs

Lunch

Time	Item	Servings	Calories	Sugar	Protein	Fat	Carbs

Dinner

Time	Item	Servings	Calories	Sugar	Protein	Fat	Carbs

Snacks

Time	Item	Servings	Calories	Sugar	Protein	Fat	Carbs

Total:

Servings	Calories	Sugar	Protein	Fat	Carbs

Date:

Breakfast

Time	Item	Servings	Calories	Sugar	Protein	Fat	Carbs

Lunch

Time	Item	Servings	Calories	Sugar	Protein	Fat	Carbs

Dinner

Time	Item	Servings	Calories	Sugar	Protein	Fat	Carbs

Snacks

Time	Item	Servings	Calories	Sugar	Protein	Fat	Carbs

Total:

Servings	Calories	Sugar	Protein	Fat	Carbs

Date:

Breakfast

Time	Item	Servings	Calories	Sugar	Protein	Fat	Carbs

Lunch

Time	Item	Servings	Calories	Sugar	Protein	Fat	Carbs

Dinner

Time	Item	Servings	Calories	Sugar	Protein	Fat	Carbs

Snacks

Time	Item	Servings	Calories	Sugar	Protein	Fat	Carbs

Total:

Servings	Calories	Sugar	Protein	Fat	Carbs

Date:

Breakfast

Time	Item	Servings	Calories	Sugar	Protein	Fat	Carbs

Lunch

Time	Item	Servings	Calories	Sugar	Protein	Fat	Carbs

Dinner

Time	Item	Servings	Calories	Sugar	Protein	Fat	Carbs

Snacks

Time	Item	Servings	Calories	Sugar	Protein	Fat	Carbs

Total:

Servings	Calories	Sugar	Protein	Fat	Carbs

Date:

Breakfast

Time	Item	Servings	Calories	Sugar	Protein	Fat	Carbs

Lunch

Time	Item	Servings	Calories	Sugar	Protein	Fat	Carbs

Dinner

Time	Item	Servings	Calories	Sugar	Protein	Fat	Carbs

Snacks

Time	Item	Servings	Calories	Sugar	Protein	Fat	Carbs

Total:

Servings	Calories	Sugar	Protein	Fat	Carbs

Date:

Breakfast

Time	Item	Servings	Calories	Sugar	Protein	Fat	Carbs

Lunch

Time	Item	Servings	Calories	Sugar	Protein	Fat	Carbs

Dinner

Time	Item	Servings	Calories	Sugar	Protein	Fat	Carbs

Snacks

Time	Item	Servings	Calories	Sugar	Protein	Fat	Carbs

Total:

Servings	Calories	Sugar	Protein	Fat	Carbs

Date:

Breakfast

Time	Item	Servings	Calories	Sugar	Protein	Fat	Carbs

Lunch

Time	Item	Servings	Calories	Sugar	Protein	Fat	Carbs

Dinner

Time	Item	Servings	Calories	Sugar	Protein	Fat	Carbs

Snacks

Time	Item	Servings	Calories	Sugar	Protein	Fat	Carbs

Total:

Servings	Calories	Sugar	Protein	Fat	Carbs

Date:

Breakfast

Time	Item	Servings	Calories	Sugar	Protein	Fat	Carbs

Lunch

Time	Item	Servings	Calories	Sugar	Protein	Fat	Carbs

Dinner

Time	Item	Servings	Calories	Sugar	Protein	Fat	Carbs

Snacks

Time	Item	Servings	Calories	Sugar	Protein	Fat	Carbs

Total:

Servings	Calories	Sugar	Protein	Fat	Carbs

Date:

Breakfast

Time	Item	Servings	Calories	Sugar	Protein	Fat	Carbs

Lunch

Time	Item	Servings	Calories	Sugar	Protein	Fat	Carbs

Dinner

Time	Item	Servings	Calories	Sugar	Protein	Fat	Carbs

Snacks

Time	Item	Servings	Calories	Sugar	Protein	Fat	Carbs

Total:

Servings	Calories	Sugar	Protein	Fat	Carbs

Date:

Breakfast

Time	Item	Servings	Calories	Sugar	Protein	Fat	Carbs

Lunch

Time	Item	Servings	Calories	Sugar	Protein	Fat	Carbs

Dinner

Time	Item	Servings	Calories	Sugar	Protein	Fat	Carbs

Snacks

Time	Item	Servings	Calories	Sugar	Protein	Fat	Carbs

Total:

Servings	Calories	Sugar	Protein	Fat	Carbs

Date:

Breakfast

Time	Item	Servings	Calories	Sugar	Protein	Fat	Carbs

Lunch

Time	Item	Servings	Calories	Sugar	Protein	Fat	Carbs

Dinner

Time	Item	Servings	Calories	Sugar	Protein	Fat	Carbs

Snacks

Time	Item	Servings	Calories	Sugar	Protein	Fat	Carbs

Total:

Servings	Calories	Sugar	Protein	Fat	Carbs

Date:

Breakfast

Time	Item	Servings	Calories	Sugar	Protein	Fat	Carbs

Lunch

Time	Item	Servings	Calories	Sugar	Protein	Fat	Carbs

Dinner

Time	Item	Servings	Calories	Sugar	Protein	Fat	Carbs

Snacks

Time	Item	Servings	Calories	Sugar	Protein	Fat	Carbs

Total:

Servings	Calories	Sugar	Protein	Fat	Carbs

Date:

Breakfast

Time	Item	Servings	Calories	Sugar	Protein	Fat	Carbs

Lunch

Time	Item	Servings	Calories	Sugar	Protein	Fat	Carbs

Dinner

Time	Item	Servings	Calories	Sugar	Protein	Fat	Carbs

Snacks

Time	Item	Servings	Calories	Sugar	Protein	Fat	Carbs

Total:

Servings	Calories	Sugar	Protein	Fat	Carbs

Date:

Breakfast

Time	Item	Servings	Calories	Sugar	Protein	Fat	Carbs

Lunch

Time	Item	Servings	Calories	Sugar	Protein	Fat	Carbs

Dinner

Time	Item	Servings	Calories	Sugar	Protein	Fat	Carbs

Snacks

Time	Item	Servings	Calories	Sugar	Protein	Fat	Carbs

Total:

Servings	Calories	Sugar	Protein	Fat	Carbs

Date:

Breakfast

Time	Item	Servings	Calories	Sugar	Protein	Fat	Carbs

Lunch

Time	Item	Servings	Calories	Sugar	Protein	Fat	Carbs

Dinner

Time	Item	Servings	Calories	Sugar	Protein	Fat	Carbs

Snacks

Time	Item	Servings	Calories	Sugar	Protein	Fat	Carbs

Total:

Servings	Calories	Sugar	Protein	Fat	Carbs

Date:

Breakfast

Time	Item	Servings	Calories	Sugar	Protein	Fat	Carbs

Lunch

Time	Item	Servings	Calories	Sugar	Protein	Fat	Carbs

Dinner

Time	Item	Servings	Calories	Sugar	Protein	Fat	Carbs

Snacks

Time	Item	Servings	Calories	Sugar	Protein	Fat	Carbs

Total:

Servings	Calories	Sugar	Protein	Fat	Carbs

Date:

Breakfast

Time	Item	Servings	Calories	Sugar	Protein	Fat	Carbs

Lunch

Time	Item	Servings	Calories	Sugar	Protein	Fat	Carbs

Dinner

Time	Item	Servings	Calories	Sugar	Protein	Fat	Carbs

Snacks

Time	Item	Servings	Calories	Sugar	Protein	Fat	Carbs

Total:

Servings	Calories	Sugar	Protein	Fat	Carbs

Date:

Breakfast

Time	Item	Servings	Calories	Sugar	Protein	Fat	Carbs

Lunch

Time	Item	Servings	Calories	Sugar	Protein	Fat	Carbs

Dinner

Time	Item	Servings	Calories	Sugar	Protein	Fat	Carbs

Snacks

Time	Item	Servings	Calories	Sugar	Protein	Fat	Carbs

Total:

Servings	Calories	Sugar	Protein	Fat	Carbs

Date:

Breakfast

Time	Item	Servings	Calories	Sugar	Protein	Fat	Carbs

Lunch

Time	Item	Servings	Calories	Sugar	Protein	Fat	Carbs

Dinner

Time	Item	Servings	Calories	Sugar	Protein	Fat	Carbs

Snacks

Time	Item	Servings	Calories	Sugar	Protein	Fat	Carbs

Total:

Servings	Calories	Sugar	Protein	Fat	Carbs

Date:

Breakfast

Time	Item	Servings	Calories	Sugar	Protein	Fat	Carbs

Lunch

Time	Item	Servings	Calories	Sugar	Protein	Fat	Carbs

Dinner

Time	Item	Servings	Calories	Sugar	Protein	Fat	Carbs

Snacks

Time	Item	Servings	Calories	Sugar	Protein	Fat	Carbs

Total:

Servings	Calories	Sugar	Protein	Fat	Carbs

Date:

Breakfast

Time	Item	Servings	Calories	Sugar	Protein	Fat	Carbs

Lunch

Time	Item	Servings	Calories	Sugar	Protein	Fat	Carbs

Dinner

Time	Item	Servings	Calories	Sugar	Protein	Fat	Carbs

Snacks

Time	Item	Servings	Calories	Sugar	Protein	Fat	Carbs

Total:

Servings	Calories	Sugar	Protein	Fat	Carbs

Date:

Breakfast

Time	Item	Servings	Calories	Sugar	Protein	Fat	Carbs

Lunch

Time	Item	Servings	Calories	Sugar	Protein	Fat	Carbs

Dinner

Time	Item	Servings	Calories	Sugar	Protein	Fat	Carbs

Snacks

Time	Item	Servings	Calories	Sugar	Protein	Fat	Carbs

Total:

Servings	Calories	Sugar	Protein	Fat	Carbs

Date:

Breakfast

Time	Item	Servings	Calories	Sugar	Protein	Fat	Carbs

Lunch

Time	Item	Servings	Calories	Sugar	Protein	Fat	Carbs

Dinner

Time	Item	Servings	Calories	Sugar	Protein	Fat	Carbs

Snacks

Time	Item	Servings	Calories	Sugar	Protein	Fat	Carbs

Total:

Servings	Calories	Sugar	Protein	Fat	Carbs

Date:

Breakfast

Time	Item	Servings	Calories	Sugar	Protein	Fat	Carbs

Lunch

Time	Item	Servings	Calories	Sugar	Protein	Fat	Carbs

Dinner

Time	Item	Servings	Calories	Sugar	Protein	Fat	Carbs

Snacks

Time	Item	Servings	Calories	Sugar	Protein	Fat	Carbs

Total:

Servings	Calories	Sugar	Protein	Fat	Carbs

Date:

Breakfast

Time	Item	Servings	Calories	Sugar	Protein	Fat	Carbs

Lunch

Time	Item	Servings	Calories	Sugar	Protein	Fat	Carbs

Dinner

Time	Item	Servings	Calories	Sugar	Protein	Fat	Carbs

Snacks

Time	Item	Servings	Calories	Sugar	Protein	Fat	Carbs

Total:

Servings	Calories	Sugar	Protein	Fat	Carbs

Date:

Breakfast

Time	Item	Servings	Calories	Sugar	Protein	Fat	Carbs

Lunch

Time	Item	Servings	Calories	Sugar	Protein	Fat	Carbs

Dinner

Time	Item	Servings	Calories	Sugar	Protein	Fat	Carbs

Snacks

Time	Item	Servings	Calories	Sugar	Protein	Fat	Carbs

Total:

Servings	Calories	Sugar	Protein	Fat	Carbs

Date:

Breakfast

Time	Item	Servings	Calories	Sugar	Protein	Fat	Carbs

Lunch

Time	Item	Servings	Calories	Sugar	Protein	Fat	Carbs

Dinner

Time	Item	Servings	Calories	Sugar	Protein	Fat	Carbs

Snacks

Time	Item	Servings	Calories	Sugar	Protein	Fat	Carbs

Total:

Servings	Calories	Sugar	Protein	Fat	Carbs

Date:

Breakfast

Time	Item	Servings	Calories	Sugar	Protein	Fat	Carbs

Lunch

Time	Item	Servings	Calories	Sugar	Protein	Fat	Carbs

Dinner

Time	Item	Servings	Calories	Sugar	Protein	Fat	Carbs

Snacks

Time	Item	Servings	Calories	Sugar	Protein	Fat	Carbs

Total:

Servings	Calories	Sugar	Protein	Fat	Carbs

Date:

Breakfast

Time	Item	Servings	Calories	Sugar	Protein	Fat	Carbs

Lunch

Time	Item	Servings	Calories	Sugar	Protein	Fat	Carbs

Dinner

Time	Item	Servings	Calories	Sugar	Protein	Fat	Carbs

Snacks

Time	Item	Servings	Calories	Sugar	Protein	Fat	Carbs

Total:

Servings	Calories	Sugar	Protein	Fat	Carbs

Date:

Breakfast

Time	Item	Servings	Calories	Sugar	Protein	Fat	Carbs

Lunch

Time	Item	Servings	Calories	Sugar	Protein	Fat	Carbs

Dinner

Time	Item	Servings	Calories	Sugar	Protein	Fat	Carbs

Snacks

Time	Item	Servings	Calories	Sugar	Protein	Fat	Carbs

Total:

Servings	Calories	Sugar	Protein	Fat	Carbs

Date:

Breakfast

Time	Item	Servings	Calories	Sugar	Protein	Fat	Carbs

Lunch

Time	Item	Servings	Calories	Sugar	Protein	Fat	Carbs

Dinner

Time	Item	Servings	Calories	Sugar	Protein	Fat	Carbs

Snacks

Time	Item	Servings	Calories	Sugar	Protein	Fat	Carbs

Total:

Servings	Calories	Sugar	Protein	Fat	Carbs

Date:

Breakfast

Time	Item	Servings	Calories	Sugar	Protein	Fat	Carbs

Lunch

Time	Item	Servings	Calories	Sugar	Protein	Fat	Carbs

Dinner

Time	Item	Servings	Calories	Sugar	Protein	Fat	Carbs

Snacks

Time	Item	Servings	Calories	Sugar	Protein	Fat	Carbs

Total:

Servings	Calories	Sugar	Protein	Fat	Carbs

Date:

Breakfast

Time	Item	Servings	Calories	Sugar	Protein	Fat	Carbs

Lunch

Time	Item	Servings	Calories	Sugar	Protein	Fat	Carbs

Dinner

Time	Item	Servings	Calories	Sugar	Protein	Fat	Carbs

Snacks

Time	Item	Servings	Calories	Sugar	Protein	Fat	Carbs

Total:

Servings	Calories	Sugar	Protein	Fat	Carbs

Date:

Breakfast

Time	Item	Servings	Calories	Sugar	Protein	Fat	Carbs

Lunch

Time	Item	Servings	Calories	Sugar	Protein	Fat	Carbs

Dinner

Time	Item	Servings	Calories	Sugar	Protein	Fat	Carbs

Snacks

Time	Item	Servings	Calories	Sugar	Protein	Fat	Carbs

Total:

Servings	Calories	Sugar	Protein	Fat	Carbs

Date:

Breakfast

Time	Item	Servings	Calories	Sugar	Protein	Fat	Carbs

Lunch

Time	Item	Servings	Calories	Sugar	Protein	Fat	Carbs

Dinner

Time	Item	Servings	Calories	Sugar	Protein	Fat	Carbs

Snacks

Time	Item	Servings	Calories	Sugar	Protein	Fat	Carbs

Total:

Servings	Calories	Sugar	Protein	Fat	Carbs

Date:

Breakfast

Time	Item	Servings	Calories	Sugar	Protein	Fat	Carbs

Lunch

Time	Item	Servings	Calories	Sugar	Protein	Fat	Carbs

Dinner

Time	Item	Servings	Calories	Sugar	Protein	Fat	Carbs

Snacks

Time	Item	Servings	Calories	Sugar	Protein	Fat	Carbs

Total:

Servings	Calories	Sugar	Protein	Fat	Carbs

Date:

Breakfast

Time	Item	Servings	Calories	Sugar	Protein	Fat	Carbs

Lunch

Time	Item	Servings	Calories	Sugar	Protein	Fat	Carbs

Dinner

Time	Item	Servings	Calories	Sugar	Protein	Fat	Carbs

Snacks

Time	Item	Servings	Calories	Sugar	Protein	Fat	Carbs

Total:

Servings	Calories	Sugar	Protein	Fat	Carbs

Date:

Breakfast

Time	Item	Servings	Calories	Sugar	Protein	Fat	Carbs

Lunch

Time	Item	Servings	Calories	Sugar	Protein	Fat	Carbs

Dinner

Time	Item	Servings	Calories	Sugar	Protein	Fat	Carbs

Snacks

Time	Item	Servings	Calories	Sugar	Protein	Fat	Carbs

Total:

Servings	Calories	Sugar	Protein	Fat	Carbs

Date:

Breakfast

Time	Item	Servings	Calories	Sugar	Protein	Fat	Carbs

Lunch

Time	Item	Servings	Calories	Sugar	Protein	Fat	Carbs

Dinner

Time	Item	Servings	Calories	Sugar	Protein	Fat	Carbs

Snacks

Time	Item	Servings	Calories	Sugar	Protein	Fat	Carbs

Total:

Servings	Calories	Sugar	Protein	Fat	Carbs

Date:

Breakfast

Time	Item	Servings	Calories	Sugar	Protein	Fat	Carbs

Lunch

Time	Item	Servings	Calories	Sugar	Protein	Fat	Carbs

Dinner

Time	Item	Servings	Calories	Sugar	Protein	Fat	Carbs

Snacks

Time	Item	Servings	Calories	Sugar	Protein	Fat	Carbs

Total:

Servings	Calories	Sugar	Protein	Fat	Carbs

Date:

Breakfast

Time	Item	Servings	Calories	Sugar	Protein	Fat	Carbs

Lunch

Time	Item	Servings	Calories	Sugar	Protein	Fat	Carbs

Dinner

Time	Item	Servings	Calories	Sugar	Protein	Fat	Carbs

Snacks

Time	Item	Servings	Calories	Sugar	Protein	Fat	Carbs

Total:

Servings	Calories	Sugar	Protein	Fat	Carbs

Date:

Breakfast

Time	Item	Servings	Calories	Sugar	Protein	Fat	Carbs

Lunch

Time	Item	Servings	Calories	Sugar	Protein	Fat	Carbs

Dinner

Time	Item	Servings	Calories	Sugar	Protein	Fat	Carbs

Snacks

Time	Item	Servings	Calories	Sugar	Protein	Fat	Carbs

Total:

Servings	Calories	Sugar	Protein	Fat	Carbs

Date:

Breakfast

Time	Item	Servings	Calories	Sugar	Protein	Fat	Carbs

Lunch

Time	Item	Servings	Calories	Sugar	Protein	Fat	Carbs

Dinner

Time	Item	Servings	Calories	Sugar	Protein	Fat	Carbs

Snacks

Time	Item	Servings	Calories	Sugar	Protein	Fat	Carbs

Total:

Servings	Calories	Sugar	Protein	Fat	Carbs

Date:

Breakfast

Time	Item	Servings	Calories	Sugar	Protein	Fat	Carbs

Lunch

Time	Item	Servings	Calories	Sugar	Protein	Fat	Carbs

Dinner

Time	Item	Servings	Calories	Sugar	Protein	Fat	Carbs

Snacks

Time	Item	Servings	Calories	Sugar	Protein	Fat	Carbs

Total:

Servings	Calories	Sugar	Protein	Fat	Carbs

Date:

Breakfast

Time	Item	Servings	Calories	Sugar	Protein	Fat	Carbs

Lunch

Time	Item	Servings	Calories	Sugar	Protein	Fat	Carbs

Dinner

Time	Item	Servings	Calories	Sugar	Protein	Fat	Carbs

Snacks

Time	Item	Servings	Calories	Sugar	Protein	Fat	Carbs

Total:

Servings	Calories	Sugar	Protein	Fat	Carbs

Date:

Breakfast

Time	Item	Servings	Calories	Sugar	Protein	Fat	Carbs

Lunch

Time	Item	Servings	Calories	Sugar	Protein	Fat	Carbs

Dinner

Time	Item	Servings	Calories	Sugar	Protein	Fat	Carbs

Snacks

Time	Item	Servings	Calories	Sugar	Protein	Fat	Carbs

Total:

Servings	Calories	Sugar	Protein	Fat	Carbs

Date:

Breakfast

Time	Item	Servings	Calories	Sugar	Protein	Fat	Carbs

Lunch

Time	Item	Servings	Calories	Sugar	Protein	Fat	Carbs

Dinner

Time	Item	Servings	Calories	Sugar	Protein	Fat	Carbs

Snacks

Time	Item	Servings	Calories	Sugar	Protein	Fat	Carbs

Total:

Servings	Calories	Sugar	Protein	Fat	Carbs

Date:

Breakfast

Time	Item	Servings	Calories	Sugar	Protein	Fat	Carbs

Lunch

Time	Item	Servings	Calories	Sugar	Protein	Fat	Carbs

Dinner

Time	Item	Servings	Calories	Sugar	Protein	Fat	Carbs

Snacks

Time	Item	Servings	Calories	Sugar	Protein	Fat	Carbs

Total:

Servings	Calories	Sugar	Protein	Fat	Carbs

Date:

Breakfast

Time	Item	Servings	Calories	Sugar	Protein	Fat	Carbs

Lunch

Time	Item	Servings	Calories	Sugar	Protein	Fat	Carbs

Dinner

Time	Item	Servings	Calories	Sugar	Protein	Fat	Carbs

Snacks

Time	Item	Servings	Calories	Sugar	Protein	Fat	Carbs

Total:

Servings	Calories	Sugar	Protein	Fat	Carbs

Date:

Breakfast

Time	Item	Servings	Calories	Sugar	Protein	Fat	Carbs

Lunch

Time	Item	Servings	Calories	Sugar	Protein	Fat	Carbs

Dinner

Time	Item	Servings	Calories	Sugar	Protein	Fat	Carbs

Snacks

Time	Item	Servings	Calories	Sugar	Protein	Fat	Carbs

Total:

Servings	Calories	Sugar	Protein	Fat	Carbs

Date:

Breakfast

Time	Item	Servings	Calories	Sugar	Protein	Fat	Carbs

Lunch

Time	Item	Servings	Calories	Sugar	Protein	Fat	Carbs

Dinner

Time	Item	Servings	Calories	Sugar	Protein	Fat	Carbs

Snacks

Time	Item	Servings	Calories	Sugar	Protein	Fat	Carbs

Total:

Servings	Calories	Sugar	Protein	Fat	Carbs

Date:

Breakfast

Time	Item	Servings	Calories	Sugar	Protein	Fat	Carbs

Lunch

Time	Item	Servings	Calories	Sugar	Protein	Fat	Carbs

Dinner

Time	Item	Servings	Calories	Sugar	Protein	Fat	Carbs

Snacks

Time	Item	Servings	Calories	Sugar	Protein	Fat	Carbs

Total:

Servings	Calories	Sugar	Protein	Fat	Carbs

Date:

Breakfast

Time	Item	Servings	Calories	Sugar	Protein	Fat	Carbs

Lunch

Time	Item	Servings	Calories	Sugar	Protein	Fat	Carbs

Dinner

Time	Item	Servings	Calories	Sugar	Protein	Fat	Carbs

Snacks

Time	Item	Servings	Calories	Sugar	Protein	Fat	Carbs

Total:

Servings	Calories	Sugar	Protein	Fat	Carbs

Date:

Breakfast

Time	Item	Servings	Calories	Sugar	Protein	Fat	Carbs

Lunch

Time	Item	Servings	Calories	Sugar	Protein	Fat	Carbs

Dinner

Time	Item	Servings	Calories	Sugar	Protein	Fat	Carbs

Snacks

Time	Item	Servings	Calories	Sugar	Protein	Fat	Carbs

Total:

Servings	Calories	Sugar	Protein	Fat	Carbs

Date:

Breakfast

Time	Item	Servings	Calories	Sugar	Protein	Fat	Carbs

Lunch

Time	Item	Servings	Calories	Sugar	Protein	Fat	Carbs

Dinner

Time	Item	Servings	Calories	Sugar	Protein	Fat	Carbs

Snacks

Time	Item	Servings	Calories	Sugar	Protein	Fat	Carbs

Total:

Servings	Calories	Sugar	Protein	Fat	Carbs

Date:

Breakfast

Time	Item	Servings	Calories	Sugar	Protein	Fat	Carbs

Lunch

Time	Item	Servings	Calories	Sugar	Protein	Fat	Carbs

Dinner

Time	Item	Servings	Calories	Sugar	Protein	Fat	Carbs

Snacks

Time	Item	Servings	Calories	Sugar	Protein	Fat	Carbs

Total:

Servings	Calories	Sugar	Protein	Fat	Carbs

Date:

Breakfast

Time	Item	Servings	Calories	Sugar	Protein	Fat	Carbs

Lunch

Time	Item	Servings	Calories	Sugar	Protein	Fat	Carbs

Dinner

Time	Item	Servings	Calories	Sugar	Protein	Fat	Carbs

Snacks

Time	Item	Servings	Calories	Sugar	Protein	Fat	Carbs

Total:

Servings	Calories	Sugar	Protein	Fat	Carbs

Date:

Breakfast

Time	Item	Servings	Calories	Sugar	Protein	Fat	Carbs

Lunch

Time	Item	Servings	Calories	Sugar	Protein	Fat	Carbs

Dinner

Time	Item	Servings	Calories	Sugar	Protein	Fat	Carbs

Snacks

Time	Item	Servings	Calories	Sugar	Protein	Fat	Carbs

Total:

Servings	Calories	Sugar	Protein	Fat	Carbs

Date:

Breakfast

Time	Item	Servings	Calories	Sugar	Protein	Fat	Carbs

Lunch

Time	Item	Servings	Calories	Sugar	Protein	Fat	Carbs

Dinner

Time	Item	Servings	Calories	Sugar	Protein	Fat	Carbs

Snacks

Time	Item	Servings	Calories	Sugar	Protein	Fat	Carbs

Total:

Servings	Calories	Sugar	Protein	Fat	Carbs

Date:

Breakfast

Time	Item	Servings	Calories	Sugar	Protein	Fat	Carbs

Lunch

Time	Item	Servings	Calories	Sugar	Protein	Fat	Carbs

Dinner

Time	Item	Servings	Calories	Sugar	Protein	Fat	Carbs

Snacks

Time	Item	Servings	Calories	Sugar	Protein	Fat	Carbs

Total:

Servings	Calories	Sugar	Protein	Fat	Carbs

Date:

Breakfast

Time	Item	Servings	Calories	Sugar	Protein	Fat	Carbs

Lunch

Time	Item	Servings	Calories	Sugar	Protein	Fat	Carbs

Dinner

Time	Item	Servings	Calories	Sugar	Protein	Fat	Carbs

Snacks

Time	Item	Servings	Calories	Sugar	Protein	Fat	Carbs

Total:

Servings	Calories	Sugar	Protein	Fat	Carbs

Date:

Breakfast

Time	Item	Servings	Calories	Sugar	Protein	Fat	Carbs

Lunch

Time	Item	Servings	Calories	Sugar	Protein	Fat	Carbs

Dinner

Time	Item	Servings	Calories	Sugar	Protein	Fat	Carbs

Snacks

Time	Item	Servings	Calories	Sugar	Protein	Fat	Carbs

Total:

Servings	Calories	Sugar	Protein	Fat	Carbs

Date:

Breakfast

Time	Item	Servings	Calories	Sugar	Protein	Fat	Carbs

Lunch

Time	Item	Servings	Calories	Sugar	Protein	Fat	Carbs

Dinner

Time	Item	Servings	Calories	Sugar	Protein	Fat	Carbs

Snacks

Time	Item	Servings	Calories	Sugar	Protein	Fat	Carbs

Total:

Servings	Calories	Sugar	Protein	Fat	Carbs

Date:

Breakfast

Time	Item	Servings	Calories	Sugar	Protein	Fat	Carbs

Lunch

Time	Item	Servings	Calories	Sugar	Protein	Fat	Carbs

Dinner

Time	Item	Servings	Calories	Sugar	Protein	Fat	Carbs

Snacks

Time	Item	Servings	Calories	Sugar	Protein	Fat	Carbs

Total:

Servings	Calories	Sugar	Protein	Fat	Carbs

Date:

Breakfast

Time	Item	Servings	Calories	Sugar	Protein	Fat	Carbs

Lunch

Time	Item	Servings	Calories	Sugar	Protein	Fat	Carbs

Dinner

Time	Item	Servings	Calories	Sugar	Protein	Fat	Carbs

Snacks

Time	Item	Servings	Calories	Sugar	Protein	Fat	Carbs

Total:

Servings	Calories	Sugar	Protein	Fat	Carbs

Date:

Breakfast

Time	Item	Servings	Calories	Sugar	Protein	Fat	Carbs

Lunch

Time	Item	Servings	Calories	Sugar	Protein	Fat	Carbs

Dinner

Time	Item	Servings	Calories	Sugar	Protein	Fat	Carbs

Snacks

Time	Item	Servings	Calories	Sugar	Protein	Fat	Carbs

Total:

Servings	Calories	Sugar	Protein	Fat	Carbs

Date:

Breakfast

Time	Item	Servings	Calories	Sugar	Protein	Fat	Carbs

Lunch

Time	Item	Servings	Calories	Sugar	Protein	Fat	Carbs

Dinner

Time	Item	Servings	Calories	Sugar	Protein	Fat	Carbs

Snacks

Time	Item	Servings	Calories	Sugar	Protein	Fat	Carbs

Total:

Servings	Calories	Sugar	Protein	Fat	Carbs

Date:

Breakfast

Time	Item	Servings	Calories	Sugar	Protein	Fat	Carbs

Lunch

Time	Item	Servings	Calories	Sugar	Protein	Fat	Carbs

Dinner

Time	Item	Servings	Calories	Sugar	Protein	Fat	Carbs

Snacks

Time	Item	Servings	Calories	Sugar	Protein	Fat	Carbs

Total:

Servings	Calories	Sugar	Protein	Fat	Carbs

Date:

Breakfast

Time	Item	Servings	Calories	Sugar	Protein	Fat	Carbs

Lunch

Time	Item	Servings	Calories	Sugar	Protein	Fat	Carbs

Dinner

Time	Item	Servings	Calories	Sugar	Protein	Fat	Carbs

Snacks

Time	Item	Servings	Calories	Sugar	Protein	Fat	Carbs

Total:

Servings	Calories	Sugar	Protein	Fat	Carbs

Date:

Breakfast

Time	Item	Servings	Calories	Sugar	Protein	Fat	Carbs

Lunch

Time	Item	Servings	Calories	Sugar	Protein	Fat	Carbs

Dinner

Time	Item	Servings	Calories	Sugar	Protein	Fat	Carbs

Snacks

Time	Item	Servings	Calories	Sugar	Protein	Fat	Carbs

Total:

Servings	Calories	Sugar	Protein	Fat	Carbs

Date:

Breakfast

Time	Item	Servings	Calories	Sugar	Protein	Fat	Carbs

Lunch

Time	Item	Servings	Calories	Sugar	Protein	Fat	Carbs

Dinner

Time	Item	Servings	Calories	Sugar	Protein	Fat	Carbs

Snacks

Time	Item	Servings	Calories	Sugar	Protein	Fat	Carbs

Total:

Servings	Calories	Sugar	Protein	Fat	Carbs

Date:

Breakfast

Time	Item	Servings	Calories	Sugar	Protein	Fat	Carbs

Lunch

Time	Item	Servings	Calories	Sugar	Protein	Fat	Carbs

Dinner

Time	Item	Servings	Calories	Sugar	Protein	Fat	Carbs

Snacks

Time	Item	Servings	Calories	Sugar	Protein	Fat	Carbs

Total:

Servings	Calories	Sugar	Protein	Fat	Carbs

Date:

Breakfast

Time	Item	Servings	Calories	Sugar	Protein	Fat	Carbs

Lunch

Time	Item	Servings	Calories	Sugar	Protein	Fat	Carbs

Dinner

Time	Item	Servings	Calories	Sugar	Protein	Fat	Carbs

Snacks

Time	Item	Servings	Calories	Sugar	Protein	Fat	Carbs

Total:

Servings	Calories	Sugar	Protein	Fat	Carbs

Date:

Breakfast

Time	Item	Servings	Calories	Sugar	Protein	Fat	Carbs

Lunch

Time	Item	Servings	Calories	Sugar	Protein	Fat	Carbs

Dinner

Time	Item	Servings	Calories	Sugar	Protein	Fat	Carbs

Snacks

Time	Item	Servings	Calories	Sugar	Protein	Fat	Carbs

Total:

Servings	Calories	Sugar	Protein	Fat	Carbs

Date:

Breakfast

Time	Item	Servings	Calories	Sugar	Protein	Fat	Carbs

Lunch

Time	Item	Servings	Calories	Sugar	Protein	Fat	Carbs

Dinner

Time	Item	Servings	Calories	Sugar	Protein	Fat	Carbs

Snacks

Time	Item	Servings	Calories	Sugar	Protein	Fat	Carbs

Total:

Servings	Calories	Sugar	Protein	Fat	Carbs

Date:

Breakfast

Time	Item	Servings	Calories	Sugar	Protein	Fat	Carbs

Lunch

Time	Item	Servings	Calories	Sugar	Protein	Fat	Carbs

Dinner

Time	Item	Servings	Calories	Sugar	Protein	Fat	Carbs

Snacks

Time	Item	Servings	Calories	Sugar	Protein	Fat	Carbs

Total:

Servings	Calories	Sugar	Protein	Fat	Carbs

Date:

Breakfast

Time	Item	Servings	Calories	Sugar	Protein	Fat	Carbs

Lunch

Time	Item	Servings	Calories	Sugar	Protein	Fat	Carbs

Dinner

Time	Item	Servings	Calories	Sugar	Protein	Fat	Carbs

Snacks

Time	Item	Servings	Calories	Sugar	Protein	Fat	Carbs

Total:

Servings	Calories	Sugar	Protein	Fat	Carbs

Date:

Breakfast

Time	Item	Servings	Calories	Sugar	Protein	Fat	Carbs

Lunch

Time	Item	Servings	Calories	Sugar	Protein	Fat	Carbs

Dinner

Time	Item	Servings	Calories	Sugar	Protein	Fat	Carbs

Snacks

Time	Item	Servings	Calories	Sugar	Protein	Fat	Carbs

Total:

Servings	Calories	Sugar	Protein	Fat	Carbs

Date:

Breakfast

Time	Item	Servings	Calories	Sugar	Protein	Fat	Carbs

Lunch

Time	Item	Servings	Calories	Sugar	Protein	Fat	Carbs

Dinner

Time	Item	Servings	Calories	Sugar	Protein	Fat	Carbs

Snacks

Time	Item	Servings	Calories	Sugar	Protein	Fat	Carbs

Total:

Servings	Calories	Sugar	Protein	Fat	Carbs

Date:

Breakfast

Time	Item	Servings	Calories	Sugar	Protein	Fat	Carbs

Lunch

Time	Item	Servings	Calories	Sugar	Protein	Fat	Carbs

Dinner

Time	Item	Servings	Calories	Sugar	Protein	Fat	Carbs

Snacks

Time	Item	Servings	Calories	Sugar	Protein	Fat	Carbs

Total:

Servings	Calories	Sugar	Protein	Fat	Carbs

Date:

Breakfast

Time	Item	Servings	Calories	Sugar	Protein	Fat	Carbs

Lunch

Time	Item	Servings	Calories	Sugar	Protein	Fat	Carbs

Dinner

Time	Item	Servings	Calories	Sugar	Protein	Fat	Carbs

Snacks

Time	Item	Servings	Calories	Sugar	Protein	Fat	Carbs

Total:

Servings	Calories	Sugar	Protein	Fat	Carbs

Date:

Breakfast

Time	Item	Servings	Calories	Sugar	Protein	Fat	Carbs

Lunch

Time	Item	Servings	Calories	Sugar	Protein	Fat	Carbs

Dinner

Time	Item	Servings	Calories	Sugar	Protein	Fat	Carbs

Snacks

Time	Item	Servings	Calories	Sugar	Protein	Fat	Carbs

Total:

Servings	Calories	Sugar	Protein	Fat	Carbs